Table of Contents

INTRODUCTION

It seems like there's a new diet invented every day. but if you've heard of the Nordic diet (also known as the Scandinavian diet), you might be curious what it's all about and if it's just another fad diet.

The Nordic diet is a health-promoting plan based on local, fresh foods in season, with an emphasis on sustainability.

The diet was created by researchers at Denmark's University of Copenhagen, along with the co-founder of the popular Danish restaurant called NOMA, which has earned the title of the "best restaurant in the world" by certain critics. It's also sometimes referred to as the new Nordic diet (NND).

It's not often that the government of a country joins forces with a well-known restauranteur to develop and promote an eating plan that's intended to improve public health. That's exactly what happened in Denmark recently with the "Nordic diet."

U.S News ranked the Nordic diet as the No. 10 best overall diet for 2022. So what is the Nordic diet, and how does it differ in terms of health benefits from the praised Mediterranean diet?

The Nordic diet meal plan is a fresh perspective on healthy Nordic and Scandinavian cuisines, which include nutrient-rich foods like fish, vegetables and whole grain breads. It has many things in common with the Mediterranean diet, but the food choices differ if you choose to follow a traditional Danish diet — such as one that includes ingredients like elk meat, herring fish, Icelandic yogurt, lingonberries, rutabaga and whole grain crisp breads.

Not only can following this diet improve your nutrient intake, but it might even have benefits for mental health, since it emphasizes eating mindfully among family and friends.

The Nordic diet also emphasizes high-quality carbohydrates: cereals, crackers, and breads made with whole-grain barley, oats, and rye. Americans may be familiar with Swedish Wasa crispbreads, most of which are made with whole grains. In Denmark, a dense, dark sourdough bread called Rugbrød is popular. These whole-grain foods provide a wealth of heart-protecting nutrients, including fiber, vitamins, minerals, and antioxidants.

Eating lots of berries is another unique aspect of the Nordic diet that may account for some of its health benefits. Research by Harvard scientists has linked eating plentiful amounts of berries (such as blueberries and strawberries) to less weight gain and a lower risk of having a heart attack. Berries are excellent sources of plant chemicals known as anthocyanins, which seem to lower blood pressure and make blood vessels more flexible. Nordic diet staples include whole-grain cereals such as rye, barley, and oats; berries and other fruits; vegetables (especially cabbage and root vegetables like potatoes and carrots); fatty fish such as salmon, mackerel, and herring; and legumes (beans and peas).

The Nordic diet incorporates foods commonly eaten by people in the Nordic countries. Several studies show that this way of eating may cause weight loss and improve health markers — at least in the short term. The Nordic diet is healthy because it replaces processed foods with whole, single-ingredient foods. It may cause short-term weight loss and some reduction in blood pressure and inflammatory markers. However, the evidence is weak and inconsistent. Generally, any diet that emphasizes whole foods instead of standard Western junk food is likely to lead to some weight loss and health improvements.

CHAPTER ONE

The History of Nordic Food Culture

Nordic food culture was birthed from a need for survival. The long, dark, frozen winters meant that it was difficult to ensure securing enough food to meet the people's nutritional needs. Thus, the foundation of the Nordic Diet is based on three factors: climate, lifestyle, and isolation. The climate, with those endless icy winters, yet bursts of sunshine in the long warm days of summer, meant that food had to be secured during the warmer months that could last over the winter. In addition, crops had to be cultivated which suited these weather patterns, such as oats, rye, beets, carrots, cabbage, and potatoes, becoming important aspects of the diet. Foods, such as herbs, berries and mushrooms were foraged during the warmers months, as well. Lifestyle also factored into food traditions, including a deep-held communion with nature and the gifts from the forest, as well as a large number of small farms dotting the landscape. Thanks to those long, dark days (in some parts of Scandinavia the sun never rises during parts of the winter), families became very isolated, having to ensure survival through their rugged tenacity. Over time, these three factors evolved into a cultural diet pattern that has been passed down through generations. Just look at these food traditions that have long been celebrated in Nordic countries: pickled herring is consumed at many holidays, crayfish parties pop up in the summertime when this shellfish is widely available in waterways, and legend has it that you should leave out a bowl of porridge at Christmas for the barn elves so that they behave themselves over the winter.

Food preservation is a great example of one of the ways climate and survival influenced the early Nordic Diet. In the mountains, milk is preserved as cheese and butter for the winter. Other examples of food preservation include fish traditions, such as dried cod, pickled herring, Norwegian lutefisk, and Icelandic fermented shark. Vegetables, such as cabbage and beets, were pickled. Berries were cooked down into concentrates to rehydrate with water later on. Breads were baked into long-lasting crispbreads, made from freshly harvested grains. Root cellars helped keep vegetables, like cabbage, carrots, potatoes, and rutabagas, edible for months. Pulses, like beans and peas, could be dried and consumed during the year in dishes, such as the weekly Pea Soup that is a classic custom in Sweden. The end result was a diet pattern rich in foraged, seasonal, local foods, such as seafood, whole grains, pulses, root and cruciferous vegetables, and fruits like apples, pears and berries.

What is Nordic Diet?

The Nordic diet was specifically designed to revolutionize Nordic cuisine and improve public health. Nutritional scientists based at Denmark's University of Copenhagen teamed up with a co-founder of the world-renowned restaurant Noma for this multi-year project. Known as the Nordic diet or New Nordic diet, it incorporates aspects of Scandinavian tradition and culture. The Nordic diet calls for a lifestyle that embraces a return to relaxed meals with friends and family, centered on seasonal, locally sourced foods, combined with concern for protecting the environment. It's recommended to consult with your primary care physician or a registered dietitian before starting this diet.

10 concepts underlying the Nordic diet:

- Eat more fruits and vegetables every day.
- Eat more whole grains.
- Include more food from the seas and lakes.
- Choose high-quality meat – but eat less meat overall.
- Seek out more food from wild landscapes.
- Use organic produce whenever possible.
- Avoid food additives.
- Base more meals on seasonal produce.
- Consume more home-cooked food.
- Produce less waste.

Low-GI foods cause a slower, lower elevation in blood sugar compared with higher-GI foods; authors say. Protein-rich foods prevent you from feeling hungry. By properly balancing nutritionally dense foods, according to the book, you can prevent weight gain or regain, reduce inflammation in the body, and lower your risk of diseases like diabetes. When choosing what to eat on the Nordic diet, you could go all-out Scandinavian: Elk meat, rapeseed oil, Icelandic yogurt, lingonberries, rutabaga and herring are just some examples of common foods in Denmark, where the diet originated. But anyone can adapt the Nordic diet because its true focus is on eating wholesome foods that are local to you.

The Nordic diet's whole food, back-to-nature approach is an attractive option for many people trying to eat in a healthier way, says Kristin Kirkpatrick, lead dietitian and manager of wellness nutrition services at the Cleveland Clinic Wellness Institute. "Despite the type of diet that still prevails in the U.S., the majority of my patients want to get back to the basics – eat as their ancestors had before processing took over the food industry."

The Nordic diet, which is based on principles that have been around for centuries, promotes a healthy way of eating by focusing on locally sourced fruits, vegetables and wild seafood.

Where's It From?

The Nordic diet, is an eating style that focuses on local, seasonal and nutritious foods sourced in the Nordic countries – Denmark, Finland, Iceland, Norway, and Sweden. The New Nordic Diet, a gastronomic interpretation of the Nordic diet, was developed in 2004 by a panel of food professionals and chefs who sought to define a new regional cuisine that would help to address growing obesity rates and unsustainable farming practices. The diet is based upon four core principles: health, gastronomic potential, sustainability, and Nordic identity. The diet has been adapted from The Baltic Sea Diet Pyramid, created by the Finnish Heart Association, the Finnish Diabetes Association and the University of Eastern Finland. The Nordic countries include Denmark, Finland, Norway, Iceland, Sweden, and Greenland. The "Nordic diet" is based on their traditional ways of eating. Like the more famous Mediterranean diet, it's not really about weight loss. Instead, it's a delicious way to eat healthy. So, what foods does it include?

Overview of Nordic diet

It might come as a surprise, but Scandinavia doesn't subsist off of meatballs and Danish butter cookies. In fact, the region that includes Norway, Sweden, Finland, Denmark, and Iceland has a centuries-old tradition of eating whole and plant-based foods. The Nordic or

Scandinavian diet refers to a modern style of eating based around these traditional foods. The diet is heavy in complex carbs, lean proteins, and healthy fats, and light on processed foods, sugar, and red meat. And it also emphasizes choosing food with a smaller environmental footprint.

A Nordic Diet is a diet that is based on plant-based foods. This type of diet has been highly studied over the past few decades and has proven beneficial for heart health, weight loss, and overall physical health. The Nordic Diet follows the principles of "mindful eating" which means eating small portions of food throughout the day and not mindless snacking. It was created by Dr. Ancel Keys in the 1950s and is still followed today by many people in Scandinavia. The Nordic diet is a low carb, high-fat, and high-protein diet that has been shown to have many health benefits. The main difference between this diet and other diets is that ketosis causes your body to store less fat because it converts them into usable energy. Even though it is possible with different diets, many health professionals say that ketosis reduces stress because you release insulin levels quickly when you are on a ketogenic diet. The Nordic Diet is a low-carbohydrate, high-protein and plant-based diet in Finland. The main difference between this diet and other diets is that ketosis makes the body store less fat because the body's reserves become fuel. Even though it is possible to get similar results with different diets, many health care providers say that ketosis lowers stress levels because insulin levels are rapidly released.

Very similar to the Mediterranean diet, the Nordic diet focuses on whole foods that are typically found in Nordic regions like Norway, Denmark and Iceland. You'll eat mostly plant-based, seasonal foods that are high in protein, complex carbohydrates and healthy fats. Think fruits (especially berries), vegetables and seafood. One difference, though, is the type of oil each diet uses. The Mediterranean diet focuses on using extra-virgin olive oil, while the Nordic diet touts canola oil. Canola oil has less saturated fat than extra-virgin olive oil and can be used in cooking and baking at a higher temperature than olive oil. It should be noted that most canola oil available in the

U.S. is processed and lacks antioxidants compared to olive oil. “Generally, both are good unsaturated, healthy anti-inflammatory oils,” says Barth. The Nordic diet encourages people to consume less sugar and twice the amount of fiber and seafood than traditional Western diets.

How Nordic Diet works

Although you don’t count calories on the Nordic diet, you’ll calculate the carb-protein ratio of your meals. Ideal meals involve a 2:1 ratio of carb grams to protein grams. For carbohydrates, start by getting familiar with low-GI foods. Most fruits and vegetables, other than potatoes, have a low glycemic index. GIs vary for other carb-containing foods such as dairy products, grains, bread, pasta, beans and legumes. Rye is a whole-grain staple in the Nordic diet. However, all breads aren’t alike: Pumpernickel and sourdough bread are low-GI, while softer, fluffy white breads aren’t. At breakfast, steel-cut oats are lower GI than instant oatmeal. Lower-fat dairy products are recommended. Protein-rich foods will help keep you satiated. In the Nordic diet, fish such as shellfish or white, fatty fishes; lean cuts of pork; veal and beef; and skinless poultry provide healthy protein. Fish – such as salmon, mackerel and sardines – provide healthy omega-3 fatty acids. Using fish as a food source is also easier on the environment than beef.

Tofu and legumes, such as lentils or beans, are good protein choices for vegetarians and meat eaters alike. Fiber comes naturally with veggies and whole grains. For extra fiber, add chia seeds to your meal. To get you started, “The Nordic Way” offers a four-week eating plan. You can go beyond the recommended portions but should only eat until you’re no longer hungry, not until you’re stuffed. A typical plate would be half-filled by veggies, fruit and berries; one-quarter low-GI carbs; and one-quarter protein-rich foods. You should eat protein at every meal. Starches such as rice and pasta are OK but in lower quantities than plant foods, lean meat and fish. Midmorning or afternoon snacks are fine. You could combine low-GI toast or crispbread with a slight splurge of dark chocolate spread, or munch on fresh fruit or nuts. You’ll prepare food from home and pack lunches as much as possible. You can visit salad bars if you favor fresh veggies over potato and pasta salads; focus on lean protein and choose low-GI sides like chickpeas. Don't forget your water bottle: You should drink water with every meal.

The Basic Principles of the Nordic Diet

The Nordic Diet is based on natural food such as vegetables, fruits, and whole grains beneficial to human health. The Basic Principles of the Nordic diet include:

- Eating breakfast every day.
- Eating dinner at night.
- Avoiding fast food.
- Eating three meals a day.
- Choosing yourself instead of processed foods.

A significant benefit of the Nordic Diet is that it is rich in omega-3 and omega-6 fatty acids. These essential nutrients have a wide range of benefits, including helping to maintain a healthy heart, reducing inflammation, and even helping prevent chronic diseases like cancer. The Nordic Diet comprises plenty of fresh, plant-based foods, including whole grains, vegetables, and fruits. It's a low-fat diet and requires you to take in more than 1,600 milligrams of calcium per day. Studies show that this type of diet can help with weight loss and can even help fight diabetes. The Nordic Diet, which has been the focus of many studies and has had positive effects on health, is now becoming more popular in the United States. The basic principles of the diet are that it consists of a whole grain-based diet with vegetables and low-fat dairy products as the primary sources of carbohydrates and fats, respectively. It also includes dried fruit, coffee, tea, herbs and spices like ginger and cinnamon, and traditional delicacies from Norway like pickled herring.

The Nordic Diet: How Did the Vikings Actually Eat?

Indeed, life in 10th century Europe was not an easy one. This was reflected in the Nordic diets that were being eaten by the Vikings at the time. While speaking about a singular Nordic diet is something we could do, it would be a grave mistake. An important aspect to understand is that trading was not as rampant as today, and highways did all but exist. Travelling between two cities by foot or horse to trade resources was not risk-free. And with that said, it was also less common compared to today.

This introduces the importance of local produce. The Nordic diet can be characterized by a few distinct similarities, but can also be very distinguishable by the area in which a particular village or town was built. We can imagine that coastal towns and villages had much more fish in their diet, as it was more abundant in their environment. Nords with settlements with nearby woods, however, could rely more heavily on wild game hunting.

In any case, let's look at the foods that the Vikings were eating in those time, and what the Nordic diet actually consisted of. We might as well start with the fact that they usually ate two meals per day, one in the mid-morning and one at dinner time.

Vegetables and fruit

Trading wasn't as rampant as it is today. This means that many vegetables and fruit we take for granted every time we visit a supermarket weren't available in those times. As such they weren't included in the traditional Nordic diet. While their climate couldn't really sustain all the possible vegetables and fruit that could have been found in Europe at the time by itself, they did eat certain vegetables and fruits that could be found in their environment. Nowadays, scientists and scholars agree that the Nordic diet of that time included turnips, spinach, peas, beets, mushrooms, leeks, onions and carrots, cabbages, mushrooms, a mixed variety of herbs, and possibly seaweeds in settlements that lived near a coastline. They also ate a variety of wild plants, many of which aren't consumed today anymore. One reason being the abundance of different foods due to globalization and capitalism, and the other being that they didn't have any other choice at the time.

An interesting example was scurvy-grass. Because this plant was high in vitamin C, it helped prevent scurvy, a vitamin C deficiency where your teeth tend to fall out. As far as fruit goes, they had to rely on foraging, this meant a number of berries such as raspberries, elderberries, hawthorn berries, cherries, strawberries etc. Plums and apples are two exceptions found in archaeological findings as well. We have fruits and vegetables covered with that.

Meat

Meat was another major source of nutrients and calories for them. Pigs, cattle, sheep, chicken, and goats were domesticated/cultivated by the Vikings; obviously different types of animals were domesticated/cultivated in different areas and were more or less abundant because of that. This gave them access to a variety of meats, as well as their organs, and other useful parts. We can imagine that they didn't really waste any of it. Knowing that, the liver and brains are two good sources of vitamins and minerals that are essential for optimal bodily functioning. Apart from that, hunting wild game and catching fish was a common practice as well. This in return helped them meet a healthy amount of protein and other nutrients found in meat. In the Nordic diet, meat wasn't a sporadic indulgence as it was in most Christian settlements at the time. Their cuisine had much more emphasis on meats that were prepared in different ways. As a side note to meat – because chicken, cattle, goats, and sheep were not a rare occurrence, eggs and dairy products weren't either. Milk, cheese, whey, and different dairy products were readily available for Vikings. This, of course, depended whether a particular household/village/settlement had animals capable of producing it and whether they had the necessary knowledge on how to do it.

But milk itself wasn't a drink that was consumed so often compared to other dairy products. Butter, whey, curds, and cheese were a more common choice. They did this because they could keep the latter edible for a longer time. Remember, there were no fridges back then.

Grains

Grains were another staple in the Nordic diet. Bread was widely consumed, and wide was its variety as well. Vikings were familiar with oats, rye, and barley. Wheat, was used as well. Furthermore, they weren't as "picky" when it came to some more exotic foodstuffs. Some archaeological diggings found that they were making flour out of acorns, tree bark, and a variety of nuts. Because they lacked the required knowledge about the nutritional value or even toxicity of some of the used foodstuffs, being slowly poisoned by their own food wasn't out of the question either. This was noted in some excavations where the researchers concluded that one particular settlement was probably mixing something into their flat bread which shortened their lifespan.

Alcohol

Speaking of grains, beer was a common drink too. This may have had some important benefits when you think about the hygiene level of their water. Water in those days had the tendency to be dirty and full of disease-spreading bacteria. So, drinking beer, which required the water to be boiled during preparation, was a safer alternative. Mead was another alcoholic alternative which was popular in Viking areas where bees were cultivated. Both of these alcoholic beverages had another practical aspect during winter times. When food was more scarce, having a constant supply of alcohol, with its rather high caloric content, was a welcome addition which enabled them to survive more easily during times of winter hardship.

That was it. As we can see, an average Viking was eating quite healthy, judging by today's standards. There were no processed foods but more importantly, it was/is a very healthy eating pattern

Differerence and Similarities between Nordic Diet and Mediterranean Diet

The Nordic diet is actually quite similar to the Mediterranean diet. Both diets encourage consumption of fruits and vegetables, whole (rather than refined) grains, fatty fish, nuts, seeds, and pulses. They also include moderate amounts of eggs and small amounts of dairy, but limit sugars and processed foods as well as red meat. There is one key difference between the diets. While the Mediterranean diet is known for its focus on olive oil, the Nordic diet promotes the consumption of canola oil.

Like olive oil, canola oil is high in heart-healthy monounsaturated fat. These fats help lower bad cholesterol (LDL) and help control blood glucose (sugar). But canola oil also contains some alpha-linolenic acid (ALA), a plant-based omega-3 fatty acid, similar to the omega-3 found in fatty fish. Omega-3 fatty acids have been shown to reduce inflammation and may help prevent chronic diseases, such as heart disease and arthritis. They may also be important for brain health and development, as well as healthy growth and development. Those familiar with the popular Mediterranean diet, will recognize quite a few similarities with the Nordic diet. Which, when you look at the geography of both places, actually makes a lot of sense. Like the Mediterranean region, Scandinavia has hundreds of miles of coastline, explaining both regions' love of seafood. This coastal proximity also makes for milder temperatures and, subsequently, better farming conditions. Which is why you'll see so many vegetables incorporated into both diets' cuisines. But the Nordic diet differs from its southern cousin in two significant ways.

They use canola oil instead of olive oil

Where the warm Mediterranean climate practically oozes with olives for oil-making, Scandinavia's climate doesn't make for prime olive farming. Instead, Sweden is home to thousands of acres of rapeseed plants — the basis for canola oil.

Note: While canola oil does make the American Heart Association's list of top better-for-you oils, research found olive oil is the better choice for managing inflammation, according to a 2014 research review.

They focus on the environmental impact

When the modern Nordic diet was developed in 2004, the creators had the environment on their minds. "The Nordic diet has a stronger emphasis on locally sourced and sustainable foods than the Mediterranean diet," says Amos. So, when eating Nordic, it's important to focus on ingredients with the lowest environmental impact, especially plant-based and locally made foods.

Is the Nordic diet right for you?

With a focus on eating locally sourced foods, following the Nordic diet can be a good way to try out local farmers markets in your area. "Many of them will have a variety of booths with farmers who harvest fruits and vegetables that are in season," says Barth. "You can also ask your local grocery store if they carry local produce and products." For some, following the Nordic diet could be challenging due to availability of local produce. It does take planning, so the time and commitment could be a challenge for some. Since produce like lingonberries and cloudberries aren't available in the U.S., you may need to modify what you eat based on what's available in your area. But whether you focus on the local aspect of sourcing foods, the Nordic diet is a good roadmap for getting yourself into a realistic eating pattern. It can even be modified for vegans and vegetarians by adding more plant-based foods into your diet. "The approach to the Nordic diet is more of a guideline that can be really sustainable for someone," says Barth. "It's just the basics and not overthinking or complicating what you eat."

How much does Nordic Diet cost?

With its emphasis on organic foods, the Nordic diet could be expensive. Unless you have access to local farmers markets and fisheries, you'll have to turn to grocery stores where fresh-from-the-garden produce and straight-from-the-water fish can be pricey.

Alternatives to the Nordic Diet

In general, the Nordic diet is a healthy diet that incorporates natural sources of proteins along with vegetables and fruit. The biggest misconception about this diet is that it's too restrictive. In reality, this diet allows for complex carbohydrates such as brown rice, quinoa and oats. The Nordic Diet, also known as the "Danish" or "Scandinavian", is a balanced diet of low-fat dairy products, fruit, vegetables, whole grains, legumes, and fish. Many experts believe that this diet is behind the nations' long-standing longevity. However, some people may find it too restrictive. The Health Benefits of the Nordic Diet The Nordic diet is a dietary pattern aiming to improve overall health and well-being by limiting the intake of sugars, saturated fats, and red meat. It is often referred to as the "healthy eating pattern for life" and contains primarily plant-based foods low in sugar and high in nutrients.

Foods to Eat on a Nordic Diet

The Nordic diet is very well known for being low in carbohydrates and fat. It is also known to be healthy due to its focus on what the body needs, such as meat, butter, fish, eggs, milk, and vegetables. It recommends eating primarily whole grains, which are high in fibre and carbohydrates that can help lower cholesterol levels while reducing heart disease risk. A Nordic diet is a nutrition plan based primarily on foods from Northern Europe. It consists mainly of plant-based foods and encourages fish, seafood, eggs, vegetables, root vegetables, berries, herbs and spices. The Nordic diet is an eating plan created in 1968 to prevent cardiovascular disease. It consists of plenty of vegetables, fruits, whole grains, and a moderate amount of protein and healthy fats. A critical difference between this diet and others is that it includes moderate amounts of dairy products such as cheese, yoghurt, and cream.

The Nordic diet encourages you to eat a lot of whole foods, particularly sourced locally and in season, including:

- Whole grains, particularly rye, barley and oats.
- Fruits, especially berries.
- Vegetables, especially root vegetables like beets, turnips and carrots.
- Fatty fish like salmon, tuna, sardines and mackerel.

- Low-fat dairy like Skyr yogurt.
- Legumes.

You should also eat the following in moderation:

- Eggs.
- Game meat like venison, rabbit and bison.

“Game meat is a good source of lean protein and is lower in saturated fat compared to red meats, which should be consumed once or twice a week,” says Barth.

Foods to avoid

Like many diets, the Nordic diet has a handful of foods to avoid or only enjoy rarely.

Rarely:

- Other red meats that aren’t game meat.
- Alcoholic beverages.

Avoid:

- Foods with added sugars.
- Processed meats like bacon and bologna.

- High salt foods like lunch meat, dried pasta and bread.
- Fast food.
- Sweetened beverages.

"Anything that's really high in saturated fat and high in sugar is inflammatory to the body," says Barth. "It causes the body to be stressed out."

Nordic diet plan guidelines

There are some basic principles that you need to follow if you decide to start with the Nordic diet. Here are the main guidelines that you need to know:

- Fill half your plate with vegetables (onions, cabbage, carrots, garlic, tomatoes, spinach, and broccoli), the rest of your plate should contain high-fiber carbs, rye bread, oats, wholewheat pasta, plus some good-quality protein like fish, or lean meat.
- Include fish in your meals 2-3 times a week, plus 1-2 portions of an oily variety like salmon or mackerel

- As a dessert eat as many berries as you can, and choose fresh ones if you can if it is not the season frozen are good too
- Help yourself to a portion or two of low-fat dairy – or a small matchbox-sized piece of cheese a day is fine

Breakfast – Almond butter sandwich with a fried egg

- 1 large egg
- 1 slice whole-grain rye or whole-rye pumpernickel bread
- 4 teaspoons almond butter

Snack – Pear with basic yogurt dip

- 1 pear
- 2/3 low-fat Greek yogurt
- 1 tablespoon Dijon mustard
- 1 tablespoon fresh lime juice
- 1 tablespoon honey
- Salt and ground black pepper

Lunch – Rye salad with berries and lemon

- 1/3 cup rye berries or pearled barley
- 1/2 cup cottage cheese
- fresh herbs
- salted water
- zest and juice of one lemon
- 1 tablespoon of canola oil
- 1 tablespoon of fresh berries

Snack – Roasted chickpeas with almonds

- 1 cup chickpeas
- 1/2 teaspoon ground cumin
- 1/2 teaspoon paprika
- 2 tablespoons coarsely chopped raw almonds
- Olive oil spray

Dinner – Chicken breast with grapes, pears, and rice

- 1/4 cup basmati rice
- 3 ounces boneless, skinless chicken breast
- 1 pear, cut into wedges
- 1 tablespoon honey

- 1-ounce pecorino Romano cheese, very thinly sliced
- Salt and freshly ground black pepper
- 10 purple grapes
- A small handful of fresh mint leaves
- 1 tablespoon chopped raw almonds

How to start eating Nordic

Ready to dive into a Nordic eating plan? Here's a sample of what a week on the diet might look like.

Monday

- Breakfast: Blueberry almond butter smoothie
- Lunch: Mushroom brown rice pilaf
- Dinner: Salmon with lemon and dill, spinach salad, and a yummy dressing

Tuesday

- Breakfast: Lemon-raspberry baked oatmeal
- Lunch: Farro salad with cauliflower and chickpeas
- Dinner: Baked honey mustard chicken, roasted brussels sprouts, brown rice

Wednesday

- Breakfast: Baked eggs with spinach
- Lunch: Tuna sandwich on whole-wheat bread, strawberries
- Dinner: Slow cooker root vegetable stew, multigrain crackers or crisps such as Wasa

Thursday

- Breakfast: Parfait with low fat skyr, raspberries, and honey
- Lunch: Roasted red pepper pizza on whole-wheat crust
- Dinner: One-pan blackened cod, sweet potatoes, and zucchini

Friday

- Breakfast: Oatmeal with blueberries
- Lunch: Turkey sandwich on rye, apple
- Dinner: Salmon salad, whole-wheat toast

Saturday

- Breakfast: Bagel with cream cheese and lox
- Lunch: Egg scramble with avocado and tomatoes, strawberries
- Dinner: Lemon pasta with chicken and peas

Sunday

- Breakfast: Whole-wheat pancakes with skyr and peaches
- Lunch: Quinoa bowl with shrimp and root vegetables
- Dinner: Mushroom-barley soup, multigrain Wasa crisps

A Closer Look at the Traditional Nordic Diet

The following foods are part of the traditional Nordic diet pattern, with an emphasis on locally produced, seasonal foods.

- Fruits and Berries: Rose hip, blueberries, lingonberries, apples, pears, and prunes
- Vegetables: Cabbage, brussels sprouts, broccoli, fennel, spinach, sugar peas, kale, mushrooms

- Root Vegetables: Onion, kohlrabi, turnips, parsnips, beetroot, and viper's grass
- Nuts: Almonds
- Legumes: Brown beans, yellow peas, and green peas
- Meat: Pasture-raised beef, lamb, and reindeer
- Poultry: Chicken and turkey
- Dairy Products: Low-fat or fermented milk and cheese
- Fish: Herring, mackerel, and salmon
- Grains/Cereals: Whole grain rye, whole grain wheat, oat bran, barley flakes, muesli, and pearled barley
- Seeds: Linseed, psyllium, and sunflower seeds
- Fats and Oils: Vegetable fat spreads, vegetable liquid margarine, sunflower oil, linseed (flaxseed) oil, and rapeseed (canola) oil
- Sweets: Jam and baked goods

What makes the Nordic diet "healthy"?

Omega-3 Fatty Acids

Omega-3 fatty acids are just about the best nutrient you can eat for your brain. The specific omega-3s that are plentiful in cold-water fish, DHA and EPA, are needed to support the integrity and function of synaptic membranes in the brain. Alpha linoleic acid (ALA) in canola oil (also heavily used in the Nordic diet) can be transformed by the body into DHA and EPA, but the conversion is rather inefficient. Getting those omega-3s from fish oil is really the best source, and typically, adults in the US don't eat nearly enough. If you prefer not to eat fish, or are opposed to eating two or more servings a week, a fish oil supplement, such as Metabolic Maintenance's Mega Omega can provide similar benefits.

Resveratrol

Like the Mediterranean diet, the Nordic diet leaves room to enjoy a moderate amount of wine with meals. Light-to-moderate wine consumption has been associated with better performance on cognitive tests after a seven-year follow-up period in healthy, older Norwegian adults. No positive effect was observed in subjects who typically drank beer or spirits, and women who abstained from alcohol completely typically saw a drop in cognitive test scores. Taken together, these results show that it is not likely the alcohol in the wine, but wine's other unique components that benefit cognition. Resveratrol, a potent antioxidant found in grapes has been shown in other studies to enhance both cerebrovascular function and cognition in post-menopausal women. Clinical trials suggest that resveratrol is able to improve cerebral blood flow, responsiveness to carbon dioxide overload, some cognitive tests, and the amount of cerebrospinal fluid level in all humans (not just women). Of course, wine is not for everyone. If for whatever reason, you are not a wine drinker, resveratrol can also be taken as a supplement in a potentially more impactful dose.

Heart-Healthy Nutrition

Other health benefits associated with the Nordic diet (aside from cognition) have been improvements to blood pressure and weight loss for individuals with obesity. It has also been proposed as a potential preventative measure against heart attacks and strokes. Eating lots of berries is a unique aspect of the Nordic diet that may account for some of these health benefits. Harvard scientists have linked eating generous amounts of berries (such as blueberries and strawberries) to less weight gain and a lower risk of having a heart attack in later years. Berries are an excellent source of plant chemicals known as anthocyanins, which have been linked to healthier blood pressure and blood vessel flexibility.

The Nordic diet also emphasizes high-quality carbohydrates: cereals, crackers, and breads made with whole-grain barley, oats, and rye. You may have tried the popular Swedish Wasa crispbreads that are distributed in the US, most of which are made with whole grains. In Denmark, a dense, dark sourdough bread called RugbrØd is popular. In Scandinavia, typically more than half the grains people consume are whole grains. In the US, only about 10% of the grains we eat are whole grains. Whole grains provide a wealth of heart-protecting nutrients, including fiber, vitamins, and minerals. The refining process (resulting in white rice or flour) leaves the same grains with very little nutritional value, and can cause dysregulated blood sugar issues.

No Junk!

Speaking of sugar issues… what's not included the diet is as important as what is included. When we regularly consume toxins and preservatives, we significantly increase the workload of our natural detoxification systems. When we stop ingesting toxic stuff, the antioxidants in our cells can focus more energy towards repairing the cellular damage that comes along with age and everyday metabolism. Sugar, and specifically refined sugar, is problematic for a long list of reasons. Your body gets all the glucose it needs from vegetables and grains. You don't need sweet treats, no matter what your sugar-addicted brain tells you. The Nordic diet suggests having one serving of fruit or fruit-sweetened food every day, but otherwise staying away from the sweet stuff.

Recipes

The Nordic diet is a healthy, tasty way to eat that has been shown to reduce the risk of heart disease and diabetes. The main difference between the Nordic diet and other diets is that the Nordic diet eliminates carbohydrates in favour of protein, healthy fats, and more vegetables. Many health professionals say that this diet reduces stress by releasing insulin levels quickly, but no studies support this claim. The Nordic diet is becoming popular for those looking to eat healthy without compromising taste. The recipes in this cookbook will help you achieve the same results. The Nordic diet is a healthy diet consisting of lean proteins, lots of fruits and vegetables, whole grains, and dairy products. This diet is characterized by low fat, high saturated fat and cholesterol content. Many cultures have used this type of diet for centuries for optimal health.

Benefits of the Nordic Diet

The Nordic Diet has many health benefits, but you'll need to be diligent about your diet if you want to reap those benefits. The key is to eat whole, unprocessed foods that contain plenty of nutrients and fibre. The Nordic diet is a diet that is rich in plant-based foods and low in animal products. The food pyramid encourages people to eat mostly fruit, vegetables, grains and legumes. Foods rich in omega-3 fatty acids include walnuts, flax seeds, salmon, herring, and mackerel and Foods rich in monounsaturated fats include avocados, almonds and olive oil. Dairy products such as milk can be included but must be consumed with care because they have been linked to obesity and heart disease. The Nordic diet is a diet that is rich in plant-based ingredients. In the Nordic countries, where these foods originate, people's health has always been very high due to this rich diet and extraordinary lifestyle. They eat high amounts of fruits, vegetables, and whole grains like rye bread and oatmeal, and all considered healthy foods. The intake of red meat is also limited. In addition to following a nutritious diet, they need to exercise regularly because their country does not have a lot of natural landscape features that can interfere with their physical fitness.

The Nordic Diet is a popular diet trend today, with many people claiming it to be the best. The Nordic Diet has many benefits that can improve your health, including weight loss and cardiovascular disease prevention. The Nordic diet typically comprises whole grains, vegetables, fruit, and berries. The benefits of the Nordic diet include weight loss, reduced risk for diabetes, heart disease and high blood pressure, increased energy levels thanks to proteins, healthy cholesterol levels and a boost in metabolism due to the presence of antioxidants and phytonutrients found in fruits and vegetables. The Nordic Nutrition Recommendations has long been a popular diet. It is rich in fruits, vegetables, whole grains, and fish and is low in red meat and dairy products. Studies have shown this diet to effectively manage diabetes, heart disease, cancer and other conditions. The Nordic Diet is a low-carb, high-fat diet that promotes weight loss, good health, and a healthy heart. Most of the foods on this diet are from local and natural resources and include many fresh fruits and vegetables. The food on this diet also emphasizes whole grains, dairy products, eggs, and seafood.

The Nordic diet is a diet that is low in carbohydrates and high in fat. The best thing about this diet is that it uses its fat stores as fuel. This means the body doesn't need to break down muscle tissue or dampen other hormones, leading to improved cognitive performance. A Nordic diet is high in plant-based foods and includes excellent fresh seafood. It also has some dairy and eggs, but carbohydrates are limited. On average, the diet is low in saturated fat and cholesterol. Cons: It's often promoted as the healthiest diet, but no solid studies support this claim. A Nordic Diet is a healthy diet primarily based on plant-based foods, and it has become increasingly popular in recent years. Though the Nordics have a much lower rate of meat consumption, they consume more fish than the average person. Many people believe the Nordic Diet can help prevent heart disease, diabetes and cancer. A Nordic diet emphasizes whole grains, vegetables, and fruits. It's a diet high in proteins and low in foods like bread, pasta, and sweets. Experts believe that it can benefit those looking to lose weight or gain muscle mass. Just make sure to eat plenty of whole-grain foods, and you'll reap the benefits of this diet without any real drawbacks. The Nordic diet gets high praise for its healthfulness! It is associated with significant improvements in metabolic health and a lower risk of many chronic diseases. Several studies have looked at the effects of the Nordic diet on health.

- Weight loss: In a study of 147 obese men and women, participants were randomly assigned to receive either the Nordic diet or an average Danish diet for 26 weeks. Participants were instructed not to purposefully restrict calories. Individuals following the Nordic diet lost 10.4 pounds (4.7 kg), while those following a typical Danish diet only lost 3.3 pounds (1.5 kg).
- Type 2 diabetes: The Nordic food index contains six foods (apples and pears, cabbage, fish, oatmeal, root vegetables, and rye bread), and was used to obtain data on adherence to a Nordic diet eating pattern. Adherence, measured on a scale from 0-6 was associated with a lower risk of type 2 diabetes. Strict adherence (a score of 5-6) conferred a reduced risk of 25% for women and 38% for men compared with poor adherence (a score of 0 points).
- Blood pressure: In the same 26-week study investigating the effects of a Nordic diet compared to a standard Danish diet on weight loss, researchers found that the Nordic diet reduced

systolic and diastolic blood pressure by 5.1 mmHg and 3.2 mmHg, respectively.

- Lipid profiles: To investigate the effects of the Nordic diet on lipid profiles, 169 individuals completed an 18-24-week intervention where they were placed on either a Nordic diet ("healthy diet) or a control diet ("the average Nordic diet"). Participants following a Nordic diet had a mild reduction in non-HDL cholesterol, as well as the LDL/HDL and Apo B/Apo A1 ratios – all of which are strong risk factors for heart disease.

Pros

- Feeling full shouldn't be an issue: To succeed on any diet nutrition experts emphasizes the importance of satiety – that satisfied feeling that you've had enough to eat. This is not going to be a problem on the Nordic diet, protein-rich foods with every meal will keep you from feeling hungry.
- Nutrition: All the major food groups are part of the Nordic diet, and the diet emphasizes whole foods

which are always healthful than the processed ones. Fruits, vegetables, and whole grains provide lots of nutrients, colorful berries offer antioxidants, fish provides omega-3 fatty acids.

- Sustainability and Environmental awareness: Four simple considerations for sustainability were used in the formulation of the Nordic diet:
- Focus on locally grown foods to minimize the transport of foodstuffs, which helps to minimize the negative impact of transportation on the environment.
- Focus on foods from organic food production. The organic production principle is based primarily on consideration for nature and biodiversity, and it is an attempt to care for the soil, biodiversity, quality, health, and the welfare of nature, including plants, animals, and humans.
- Focus on composing a proportion of the diet from foods sourced from the wild countryside, encouraging biodiversity, and minimizing the use of fertilizers and pesticides.

- Focus on minimizing waste and utilizing all of every food purchased.

Cons

- Time-consuming: Processed foods are not allowed, which means the majority of what you eat should be prepared at home. Also, the diet's creators recommend meals to be consumed in a leisurely, mindful way which some people may find challenging if they are short of time. Routinely preparing and sitting down for homemade meals requires a significant lifestyle commitment.
- Expensive: Organic products and fish can be costly even if you live in a place where the seafood is plentiful or there are lots of organic farms.

Risks and Side Effects

Generally speaking, this NND diet is very safe for people of all ages to follow. If you have a history of chronic disease and take medications, it's best to get your doctor's opinion before altering your diet or starting a new protocol.

That being said, there are little risks associated with this plan, assuming you aim for balanced meals that include a variety of food groups.

CHAPTER TWO

Nordic Diet Recipes

Tequila-Lime Chicken

Recipe Summary

Prep: 10 mins

Cook: 35 mins

Additional: 1 hr

Total: 1 hr 45 mins

Servings: 4

Yield: 4 servings

Ingredients

- 3 skinless, boneless chicken breasts
- ½ cup tequila
- 1 lime, zested and juiced
- ¼ teaspoon garlic powder, divided
- ¼ teaspoon chili powder, divided

- 3 ounces shredded Mexican-style cheese blend

Directions

Step 1

Arrange chicken breasts in a baking dish; add tequila and juice of 1/2 a lime. Sprinkle 1/2 of the lime zest, 1/2 of the garlic powder, and 1/2 of the chili powder over the chicken. Cover dish with plastic wrap and marinate in the refrigerator for 30 minutes.

Step 2

Turn chicken breasts; sprinkle remaining lime juice, lime zest, garlic powder, and chili powder on top. Cover again and marinate in the refrigerator for another 30 minutes.

Step 3

Preheat the oven to 425 degrees F (220 degrees C). Uncover baking dish and discard tequila-lime marinade.

Step 4

Bake chicken in the preheated oven for 25 minutes. Sprinkle Mexican-style cheese over the chicken and continue to bake until the chicken is no longer pink in the center and the juices run clear, about 10 minutes more. An instant-read thermometer inserted into the center should read at least 165 degrees F (74 degrees C).

Nutrition Facts

Per Serving: 244 calories; protein 22.5g; carbohydrates 1.7g; fat 8.8g; cholesterol 68.8mg; sodium 207mg.

Tequila Lime Burgers

Recipe Summary

Prep: 10 mins

Cook: 20 mins

Total: 30 mins

Servings: 8

Yield: 8 burgers

Ingredients

- 2 pounds ground beef

- ¼ cup steak sauce
- ¼ cup Worcestershire sauce
- 2 tablespoons Montreal steak seasoning
- 2 tablespoons tequila
- 2 tablespoons fresh lime juice
- 1 teaspoon lime zest

Directions

Step 1

Preheat an outdoor grill for high heat and lightly oil grate.

Step 2

Mix together the ground beef, steak sauce, Worcestershire sauce, Montreal seasoning, tequila, lime juice, and lime zest in a large bowl until evenly combined. Form 8 patties from the mixture.

Step 3

Cook patties on preheated grill to desired doneness, 7 to 10 minutes each side for well done.

Nutrition Facts

Per Serving: 225 calories; protein 19.2g; carbohydrates 4g; fat 13.4g; cholesterol 69mg; sodium 950.7mg.

Marinated Fajita Chicken

Recipe Summary

Prep: 10 mins

Cook: 35 mins

Additional: 8 hrs

Total: 8 hrs 45 mins

Servings: 4

Yield: 4 servings

Ingredients

- 1 cup lime juice
- 4 ½ teaspoons olive oil
- 2 cloves garlic, crushed
- ½ teaspoon ground cumin
- ½ teaspoon chili powder

- ¼ teaspoon salt
- ¼ teaspoon red pepper flakes
- 5 skinless, boneless chicken breast halves

Directions

Step 1

Whisk together the lime juice, olive oil, garlic, ground cumin, chili powder, salt, and red pepper flakes in a bowl; pour into a large resealable plastic bag.

Step 2

Put the chicken breasts into the bag, coat with the marinade, squeeze out excess air, and seal the bag.

Step 3

Marinate in the refrigerator for 8 hours to overnight.

Step 4

Preheat the oven to 375 degrees F (190 degrees C).

Step 5

Remove the chicken from the marinade and shake off excess. Discard remaining marinade. Arrange chicken breasts in a baking dish.

Step 6

Bake chicken breasts in preheated oven until no longer pink in the center and the juices run clear, about 35 minutes. An instant-read thermometer inserted into the center should read at least 165 degrees F (74 degrees C).

Step 7

Shred chicken breasts with two forks to desired texture.

Nutrition Facts

Per Serving: 242 calories; protein 26.5g; carbohydrates 6.1g; fat 12.6g; cholesterol 71.3mg; sodium 209.7mg.

Chocolate-y Iced Mocha

Recipe Summary

Prep: 5 mins

Cook: 1 min

Total: 6 mins

Servings: 1

Yield: 1 serving

Ingredients

- 1 ¼ cups cold coffee, divided
- 1 envelope low-calorie hot cocoa mix
- ice cubes, or as needed
- ½ cup unsweetened almond milk
- 2 tablespoons sugar-free chocolate syrup, or more to taste

Directions

Step 1

Heat 1/4 cup coffee in microwave in a mug until warmed, about 30 seconds. Stir cocoa mix into the coffee until dissolved.

Step 2

Fill a large glass with ice cubes. Pour 1 cup cold coffee and almond milk over the ice cubes; stir the cocoa mixture and chocolate syrup into the coffee and almond milk.

Nutrition Facts

Per Serving: 105 calories; protein 5.2g; carbohydrates 16.7g; fat 1.8g; cholesterol 2.9mg; sodium 255.3mg.

Iced Mocha Cola

Recipe Summary

Prep: 5 mins

Total: 5 mins

Servings: 1

Yield: 1 serving

Ingredients

- ice, or as needed
- 1 tablespoon instant coffee granules
- 1 (12 fluid ounce) can or bottle cola-flavored carbonated beverage, or as needed.

- 1 ½ fluid ounces half-and-half

Directions

Step 1

Fill a tall glass with ice. Add instant coffee granules. Slowly pour cola into the glass. Gently stir half-and-half into the cola to integrate.

Nutrition Facts

Per Serving: 217 calories; protein 1.6g; carbohydrates 41.5g; fat 5.2g; cholesterol 16.8mg; sodium 41.7mg.

Sugar-Free Cream Cheese Frosting

Recipe Summary

Prep: 5 mins

Total: 5 mins

Servings: 12

Yield: 12 servings

Ingredients

- 1 (8 ounce) package reduced-fat cream cheese, softened
- ½ cup granular sucrolose sweetener or more to taste
- 1 (8 ounce) container frozen whipped topping, thawed
- 1 teaspoon vanilla extract

Directions

Step 1

Beat cream cheese and sucralose sweetener together in a bowl using an electric mixer until smooth and creamy; stir in whipped topping and vanilla extract until smooth.

Nutrition Facts

Per Serving: 104 calories; protein 2.2g; carbohydrates 5.7g; fat 8.1g; cholesterol 10.6mg; sodium 60.7mg.

Creamy Cream Cheese Frosting

Recipe Summary

Prep: 10 mins

Total: 10 mins

Servings: 12

Yield: 1 frosting for 1 cake

Ingredients

- 1 (3 ounce) package cream cheese
- 1 ¾ cups confectioners' sugar
- 1 (8 ounce) container frozen whipped topping, thawed

Directions

Step 1

In a large bowl, beat cream cheese and sugar until smooth. Fold in whipped topping.

Nutrition Facts

Per Serving: 155 calories; protein 0.8g; carbohydrates 22.7g; fat 7.2g; cholesterol 7.8mg; sodium 25.8mg.

Keto-Friendly Bread

Recipe Summary

Prep: 15 mins

Cook: 35 mins

Additional: 10 mins

Total: 1 hr

Servings: 8

Yield: 8 servings

Ingredients

- cooking spray
- 6 eggs, separated
- ¼ teaspoon cream of tartar
- 6 tablespoons coconut flour
- 6 tablespoons almond flour
- 2 tablespoons arrowroot powder
- 1 teaspoon gluten-free baking powder
- ½ teaspoon kosher salt
- ¼ cup coconut oil, melted and cooled

- 1 tablespoon honey

Directions

Step 1

Preheat the oven to 350 degrees F (175 degrees C). Spray a 4x8-inch loaf pan with cooking spray.

Step 2

Beat egg whites in a glass, metal, or ceramic bowl until foamy. Gradually add cream of tartar, continuing to beat until soft peaks form. Set aside.

Step 3

Combine coconut flour, almond flour, arrowroot powder, baking powder, and salt in a bowl and mix well.

Step 4

Beat egg yolks using an electric mixer in a bowl until thick. Add coconut oil and honey; mix well. Add flour mixture and stir until well combined. Fold in 1/4 of the beaten egg whites until incorporated. Add 1/2 the remaining egg whites and gently fold until only small amounts of egg whites are visible. Repeat with remaining egg whites. Pour mixture into prepared loaf pan and smooth the top.

Step 5

Bake in the preheated oven until nicely golden brown on top, about 35 minutes. Remove from oven, set on a wire rack, and let cool for 10 minutes. Run a knife around the sides, tip out bread onto a rack, and let cool completely.

Cook's Note:

The bread can be flavored in any way you like, for example, with a little artificial sweetener and almond, orange, or lemon extract for a breakfast or dessert treat, or herbs for a savory side.

Nutrition Facts

Per Serving: 181 calories; protein 6.3g; carbohydrates 9.8g; fat 13.7g; cholesterol 122.8mg; sodium 227.3mg.

Best Keto Bread

Recipe Summary

Prep: 15 mins

Cook: 45 mins

Total: 1 hr

Servings: 12

Yield: 1 loaf

Ingredients

- cooking spray
- 7 eggs, at room temperature
- ½ cup butter, melted and cooled
- 2 tablespoons olive oil
- 2 cups blanched almond flour
- 1 teaspoon baking powder
- ½ teaspoon xanthan gum
- ½ teaspoon sea salt

Directions

Step 1

Preheat the oven to 350 degrees F (175 degrees C). Grease a silicone loaf pan with cooking spray.

Step 2

Whisk eggs in a bowl until smooth and creamy, about 3 minutes. Add melted butter and olive oil; mix until well combined.

Step 3

Combine almond flour, baking powder, xanthan gum, and salt in a separate bowl; mix well. Add gradually to the egg mixture, mixing well until a thick batter is formed.

Step 4

Pour batter into the prepared pan and smooth the top with a spatula.

Step 5

Bake in the preheated oven until a toothpick inserted into the center comes out clean, about 45 minutes.

Cook's Note:

Make sure the eggs are at room temperature; this will make the bread airy and taste better.

Nutrition Facts

Per Serving: 247 calories; protein 7.7g; carbohydrates 4.9g; fat 22.8g; cholesterol 115.8mg; sodium 209.3mg.

Whole Wheat Oatmeal Strawberry Blueberry Muffins

Recipe Summary

Prep: 20 mins

Cook: 18 mins

Total: 38 mins

Servings: 12

Yield: 12 servings

Ingredients

- 1 cup whole wheat flour
- 1 cup oats
- ½ cup white sugar

- 2 teaspoons baking powder
- ½ teaspoon baking soda
- ½ teaspoon salt
- 1 cup milk
- ¼ cup vegetable oil
- 1 egg
- 1 teaspoon vanilla extract
- 2 cups diced strawberries
- 1 cup fresh blueberries

Directions

Step 1

Preheat oven to 425 degrees F (220 degrees C). Grease muffin cups or line with paper muffin liners.

Step 2

Mix flour, oats, sugar, baking powder, baking soda, and salt together in a bowl. Combine milk, vegetable oil, egg, and vanilla extract in a separate bowl.

Step 3

Stir milk mixture into flour mixture until batter is combined. Fold in strawberries and blueberries. Spoon batter into prepared muffin pan until full.

Step 4

Bake in preheated oven until a toothpick inserted into the center comes out clean, 18 to 22 minutes.

Nutrition Facts

Per Serving: 164 calories; protein 3.7g; carbohydrates 25.1g; fat 6.1g; cholesterol 15.3mg; sodium 245.4mg.

Keto Buns

Recipe Summary

Prep: 20 mins

Cook: 50 mins

Total: 1 hr 10 mins

Servings: 8

Yield: 8 servings

Ingredients

- ⅔ cup finely ground almonds
- ¼ cup coconut flour
- ⅓ cup flaxseed meal
- 3 tablespoons psyllium husk powder
- 1 teaspoon baking powder
- 1 teaspoon onion powder
- ½ teaspoon salt, or to taste
- 1 tablespoon sesame seeds, or as desired
- 3 egg whites
- 1 egg
- 1 teaspoon apple cider vinegar
- 1 cup lukewarm water

Directions

Step 1

Preheat the oven to 350 degrees F (175 degrees C).

Step 2

Combine ground almonds, coconut flour, flaxseed meal, psyllium husk powder, baking powder, onion powder, and salt in a bowl.

Step 3

Combine egg whites and egg in a separate bowl. Add vinegar and mix well. Add wet ingredients to the bowl with the flour mixture and mix well. Add water. Blend using an electric mixer until a dough forms.

Step 4

Divide dough into 8 equal parts and place on a baking sheet. Shape into buns and sprinkle with sesame seeds.

Step 5

Bake in the preheated oven until golden brown, about 50 minutes.

Cook's Note:

Do not substitute fresh egg whites with liquid egg whites from a carton.

Nutrition Facts

Per Serving: 130 calories; protein 6g; carbohydrates 9.3g; fat 8.8g; cholesterol 23.3mg; sodium 239.8mg.

Vegan Strawberry Muffins

Recipe Summary

Prep: 20 mins

Cook: 30 mins

Additional: 5 mins

Total: 55 mins

Servings: 24

Yield: 2 dozen muffins

Ingredients

- cooking spray
- 2 cups soy milk
- ¾ cup unsweetened applesauce
- 2 tablespoons white vinegar
- 4 teaspoons vanilla extract

- 2 ½ cups white whole wheat flour
- 2 cups turbinado sugar
- 1 cup whole wheat flour
- 1 cup rolled oats
- 2 teaspoons baking soda
- 1 teaspoon salt
- 1 cup diced strawberries

Directions

Step 1

Preheat oven to 350 degrees F (175 degrees C). Grease 2 muffin tins with cooking spray.

Step 2

Mix soy milk, applesauce, vinegar, and vanilla extract together in a bowl.

Step 3

Sift white whole wheat flour and whole wheat flour together into a separate bowl. Add oats, baking soda, and salt in a separate bowl. Mix in soy milk mixture until smooth. Let batter sit for 5 minutes.

strawberries into the batter. Fill muffin tins 2/3 full batter.

Step 5

Bake in the preheated oven until muffin tops are brown and sides pull away from the tin, 30 to 40 minutes.

Nutrition Facts

Per Serving: 155 calories; protein 3.5g; carbohydrates 34.5g; fat 0.9g; sodium 219.2mg.

Diet Soup

Recipe Summary

Prep: 20 mins

Cook: 30 mins

Total: 50 mins

Servings: 8

Yield: 8 servings

Ingredients

- 1 medium head cabbage, chopped
- 1 onion, chopped
- 3 large carrots, chopped
- 3 stalks celery, chopped
- 3 tomatoes, chopped
- 16 ounces frozen green beans
- 2 (1 ounce) packages dry onion soup mix
- 6 cups water

Directions

Step 1

Combine water, soup mix, and vegetables in a large stock pot. Bring to a boil. Reduce heat, and simmer until the vegetables are tender.

Nutrition Facts

Per Serving: 94 calories; protein 3.6g; carbohydrates 21g; fat 0.5g; sodium 672.9mg.

Kitchen Sink Soup

Recipe Summary

Prep: 20 mins

Cook: 30 mins

Total: 50 mins

Servings: 10

Yield: 10 servings

Ingredients

- 10 cups chicken broth
- 2 potatoes, cubed
- 2 carrots, sliced
- 2 stalks celery, diced
- 5 fresh mushrooms, sliced
- 1 green bell pepper, chopped
- 1 fresh broccoli, chopped
- 4 cups cauliflower florets
- 1 parsnip, sliced
- 1 onion, chopped

- 1 cup green peas
- 1 cup cut green beans, drained
- 1 cup wax beans, drained
- ½ cup cooked chickpeas
- ½ cup cooked navy beans
- salt and pepper to taste
- 1 teaspoon dried parsley

Directions

Step 1

In a large stockpot, combine all the ingredients and cook over medium heat partially covered for about 30 minutes or until all the vegetables are tender. Serve hot with buttered biscuits.

Nutrition Facts

Per Serving: 160 calories; protein 10.3g; carbohydrates 26.3g; fat 1.9g; sodium 1008.1mg.

Chocolate Chip Cookies for Special Diets

Recipe Summary

Prep: 15 mins

Cook: 12 mins

Additional: 23 mins

Total: 50 mins

Servings: 48

Yield: 4 dozen

Ingredients

- ½ cup butter, softened
- ¾ cup granulated artificial sweetener
- 2 tablespoons water
- ½ teaspoon vanilla extract
- 1 egg, beaten
- 1 ⅛ cups all-purpose flour
- ½ teaspoon baking soda
- ½ teaspoon salt
- ½ cup semisweet chocolate chips
- ½ cup chopped pecans

Directions

Step 1

Preheat oven to 375 degrees F (190 degrees C).

Step 2

In a medium bowl, cream together the butter and sugar substitute. Mix in water, vanilla, and egg. Sift together the flour, baking soda, and salt; stir into the creamed mixture. Mix in the chocolate chips and pecans. Drop cookies by heaping teaspoonfuls onto a cookie sheet.

Step 3

Bake in the preheated oven for 10 to 12 minutes. Remove from cookie sheets to cool on wire racks. These cookies freeze well.

Nutrition Facts

Per Serving: 60 calories; protein 4.2g; carbohydrates 3.5g; fat 3.4g; cholesterol 9mg; sodium 53.8mg.

Balalaika

Recipe Summary

Prep: 1 min

Total: 1 min

Servings: 1

Yield: 1 serving

Ingredients

- 1 fluid ounce vodka
- ½ fluid ounce cointreau
- 1 fluid ounce lemon juice
- 1 slice lemon, for garnish

Directions

Step 1

Pour the vodka and Cointreau in a highball glass with ice. Add enough lemon juice to reach the halfway point of the glass, or to taste. Garnish with a slice of lemon on the outside of glass.

Nutrition Facts

Per Serving: 124 calories; protein 0.3g; carbohydrates 10.2g; fat 0.1g; cholesterol 0mg; sodium 1.9mg.

Peach Cosmos

Recipe Summary

Prep: 5 mins

Total: 5 mins

Servings: 1

Yield: 1 cocktail

Ingredients

- ice cubes
- 2 fluid ounces peach-flavored vodka
- 1 fluid ounce cranberry juice
- ½ fluid ounce orange liqueur, such as Triple Sec
- 1 wedge fresh lime
- 1 twist lemon zest

Directions

Step 1

Fill a cocktail shaker with ice. Add peach vodka, cranberry juice, orange liqueur, and a squeeze of lime juice. Cover and shake vigorously until completely chilled, about 1 minute.

Step 2

Strain into a chilled wine glass. Garnish with lemon twist.

Nutrition Facts

Per Serving: 193 calories; protein 0.1g; carbohydrates 11.3g; fat 0.1g; sodium 1.8mg.

Lemon Drop II

Recipe Summary

Prep: 2 mins

Total: 2 mins

Servings: 4

Yield: 4 servings

Ingredients

- 4 fluid ounces citron vodka
- 2 teaspoons lemon juice
- 4 fluid ounces triple sec liqueur
- 4 maraschino cherries

Directions

Step 1

Place one maraschino cherry into each of 4 shot glasses or cordial glasses. Combine the vodka, lemon juice and triple sec in a chilled cocktail shaker. Shake then pour over maraschino cherries in the glasses.

Nutrition Facts

Per Serving: 171 calories; protein 0g; carbohydrates 13.5g; fat 0.1g; cholesterol 0mg; sodium 2.3mg.

Juicy Slow Cooker Chicken Breast for Any Diet

Recipe Summary

Prep: 10 mins

Cook: 6 hrs

Total: 6 hrs 10 mins

Servings: 4

Yield: 4 servings

Ingredients

- 1 pound skinless, boneless chicken breast halves
- 1 (14.5 ounce) can petite diced tomatoes
- ¼ onion, chopped (Optional)
- 1 teaspoon Italian seasoning (Optional)
- 1 clove garlic, minced (Optional)

Directions

Step 1

Arrange chicken in a slow cooker. Pour tomatoes over chicken; add onion, Italian seasoning, and garlic.

Step 2

Cook on Low for 6 to 8 hours.

Cook's Note:

You can use any type of herb in place of the Italian seasoning.

Nutrition Facts

Per Serving: 144 calories; protein 23.1g; carbohydrates 5.2g; fat 2.4g; cholesterol 58.5mg; sodium 208mg.

Balsamic Marinated Chicken Breasts

Recipe Summary

Prep: 15 mins

Cook: 40 mins

Additional: 30 mins

Total: 1 hr 25 mins

Servings: 4

Yield: 4 chicken breasts

Ingredients

- ¾ cup balsamic vinegar
- ½ cup water

- 1 teaspoon dried minced onion
- ½ teaspoon crushed red pepper flakes
- ½ teaspoon dried minced garlic
- ¼ teaspoon salt
- ¼ teaspoon ground black pepper
- ¼ teaspoon paprika
- ¼ teaspoon crushed dried rosemary
- ¼ teaspoon dried parsley flakes
- ¼ teaspoon chili powder
- ⅛ teaspoon dried oregano
- 4 (6 ounce) skinless, boneless chicken breast halves

Directions

Step 1

Whisk together the balsamic vinegar, water, onion, red pepper flakes, garlic, salt, pepper, paprika, rosemary, parsley, chili powder, and oregano in a bowl, and pour into a resealable plastic bag. Add the chicken breasts, coat with the marinade, squeeze out excess air, and seal the bag. Marinate in the refrigerator 30 minutes to overnight.

Step 2

Preheat oven to 400 degrees F (200 degrees C). Line a baking sheet with aluminum foil, or lightly grease a broiler pan. Remove the chicken breasts from the marinade, and shake off excess. Discard the remaining marinade, and place the chicken breasts onto the baking sheet.

Step 3

Bake in the preheated oven until the chicken breasts are golden brown and no longer pink in the center, 30 to 40 minutes. An instant-read thermometer inserted into the center should reach 165 degrees F (74 degrees C).

Nutrition Facts

Per Serving: 222 calories; protein 35.7g; carbohydrates 8g; fat 4.3g; cholesterol 96.9mg; sodium 244.3mg.

Bacon and Feta Stuffed Chicken Breast

Recipe Summary

Prep: 10 mins

Cook: 3 hrs

Total: 3 hrs 10 mins

Servings: 8

Yield: 8 stuffed chicken breasts

Ingredients

- 8 slices bacon
- ½ cup crumbled feta
- 8 skinless, boneless chicken breast halves
- 4 (14.5 ounce) cans diced tomatoes
- 2 tablespoons chopped fresh basil

Directions

Step 1

Place the bacon in a large, deep skillet, and cook over medium-high heat, turning occasionally, until evenly browned, about 10 minutes. Drain the bacon slices on a paper towel-lined plate. Let cool, then crumble into small pieces.

Step 2

Mix bacon and feta together in small bowl.

Step 3

Cut a 2 to 3 inch slit lengthwise in the side of the chicken breast creating a pocket, and fill with mixture. Secure shut with toothpicks.

Step 4

Place chicken in slow cooker, then add tomatoes and basil.

Step 5

Cook on High until chicken is no longer pink in the middle, about three hours.

Nutrition Facts

Per Serving: 246 calories; protein 33.7g; carbohydrates 7.2g; fat 7.3g; cholesterol 86.8mg; sodium 710.9mg.

Watermelon Fruit Bowl

Recipe Summary

All of your favorite fruits, lightly sweetened, served in a watermelon 'bowl'.

Prep:30 mins

Cook:5 mins

Additional:15 mins

Total:50 mins

Servings:20

Yield:20 servings

Ingredients

1 large watermelon

1 cantaloupe, halved and seeded

1 honeydew melon, halved and seeded

2 (15 ounce) cans mandarin oranges, drained

2 (20 ounce) cans pineapple chunks, drained

2 cups halved fresh strawberries

2 cups seedless grapes

½ cup water

¼ cup white sugar

2 tablespoons grated lemon zest

Directions

Step 1

With a large, sharp knife, remove the top 1/4 section of the watermelon. With a melon baller, scoop flesh from inside of watermelon, removing as many seeds as possible. Leave 1/2 inch of flesh inside the shell of the watermelon. Scoop cantaloupe and honeydew in the same manner, removing as much flesh as possible, and discarding the rinds. Refrigerate fruits separatcly until ready to assemble.

Step 2

In a small saucepan over medium-high heat, bring water and sugar to a boil. Remove from heat, and continue stirring until sugar has completely dissolved. Add lemon zest, and set aside to cool

Step 3

To serve, place watermelon balls, cantaloupe, honeydew, oranges, pineapple, strawberries, and grapes, in a large mixing bowl. Pour syrup over, and toss thoroughly. Transfer mixture to watermelon bowl, and serve. Set aside any fruit mixture that will not fit. There will be enough fruit to refill the bowl.

Nutrition Facts

Per Serving: 179 calories; protein 2.8g; carbohydrates 45.4g; fat 0.7g; sodium 23.4mg.

Pears and Dried Fruits in a Tagine

Recipe Summary

Pears and other dried fruits with lemon and honey cooked in a tagine.

Prep: 10 mins

Cook: 40 mins

Additional: 10 mins

Total: 1 hr

Servings:4

Yield:4 servings

Ingredients

1 organic lemon

2 tablespoons honey

1 (3 inch) cinnamon stick

1 vanilla bean, cut in half lengthwise

2 pears - peeled, cored, and quartered

8 pitted prunes

8 dried apricots

¼ cup blanched whole almonds

⅛ cup pine nuts

Directions

Step 1

Preheat the oven to 375 degrees F (190 degrees C).

Step 2

Wash lemon and remove peel with a knife, trying to keep it in one long string. Squeeze juice from 1/2 of the lemon into a small saucepan. Add honey, cinnamon stick, and vanilla bean. Bring to a boil, then lower heat and simmer until fragrant and syrupy, about 5 minutes

Step 3

Arrange pears, core-sides up, in a tagine. Add prunes, apricots, almonds, and lemon peel around the pears and on top if necessary. Pour lemon juice mixture over top allowing cinnamon stick and vanilla bean halves to fall into the tagine. Cover

Step 4

Cook in the preheated oven for 20 minutes. Remove from the oven and take off the cover, allowing any condensation to fall back into the tagine. Turn pears over and add pine nuts. Replace the cover and cook for 10 minutes. Turn the oven off, and allow the tagine to sit in the hot oven until sauce thickens a bit, about 10 minutes. Serve.

Cook's Note:

You can use agave in place of honey

Nutrition Facts

Per Serving: 266 calories; protein 4.7g; carbohydrates 54.2g; fat 7g; sodium 5.1mg.

Fruit Salad

Recipe Summary

Prep:20 mins

Additional:8 hrs

Total:8 hrs 20 mins

Servings:16

Yield:16 servings

Ingredients

2 cups green grapes

2 cups sliced strawberries

2 cups sliced peaches

2 cups orange segments

1 cup peeled sliced kiwi

½ cup orange juice

½ cup orange-flavored liqueur

2 tablespoons white sugar

Directions

Step 1

Mix grapes, strawberries, peaches, orange segments, and kiwi in a large bowl.

Step 2

Whisk orange juice, orange-flavored liqueur, and sugar together in a bowl until sugar dissolves; gently stir into fruit until evenly coated. Cover bowl with plastic wrap and refrigerate up to 8 hours.

Cook's Note:

The number of servings is approximate. I have served this Christmas morning as well as at Easter as an accompaniment for baked ham. It is beautiful in a trifle bowl on any buffet table.

Nutrition Facts

Per Serving: 88 calories; protein 0.9g; carbohydrates 18.7g; fat 0.3g; sodium 2.7mg.

CONCLUSION

“The Nordic diet is a healthy dietary pattern that shares many elements with the Mediterranean diet,” says Dr. Frank Hu, professor of nutrition at the Harvard T.H. Chan School of Public Health. The Mediterranean diet — widely considered the best eating pattern for preventing heart disease — also emphasizes plant-based foods. Both diets include moderate amounts of fish, eggs, and small amounts of dairy, but limit processed foods, sweets, and red meat. While the Mediterranean diet includes olive oil, the Nordic diet favors rapeseed oil (also known as canola oil). Like olive oil, canola oil is high in healthy monounsatured fat. But it also contains some alpha-linolenic acid, a plant-based omega-3 fatty acid similar to the omega-3 fatty acids found in fish. Of course, fatty fish — the richest dietary source of omega-3s — play a role in both Nordic and Mediterranean diets (try for two to three servings a week).

www.ingramcontent.com/pod-product-compliance
Lightning Source LLC
LaVergne TN
LVHW010115170826
845678LV00012B/2415

* 9 7 9 8 8 4 8 5 6 9 1 4 8 *